Your Peace Diet:
Using Yoga Principles to Reduce Stress and Anxiety

Lakshmi Gosyne

Copyright © 2011 Lakshmi Gosyne

All rights reserved.

ISBN-13:978-1461197249
ISBN-10:1461197244

This book is a general educational health-related information product. As an express condition to reading to this book, you understand and agree to the following terms. The book's content is not a substitute for direct, personal, professional medical care and diagnosis. None of the exercises or treatments (including products and services) mentioned in this book should be performed or otherwise used without clearance from your physician or health care provider.

There may be risks associated with participating in activities or using products mentioned in this book for people in poor health or with previously existing physical or mental health conditions. Because these risks exist, you will not use such products or participate in such activities if you are in poor health or have a previously existing mental or physical condition. If you choose to participate in these risks, you do so of your own free will and accord, knowingly and voluntarily assuming all risks associated with such activities.

DEDICATION

To PHSA and JS

CONTENTS

	Acknowledgments	i
1	Chapter One: Yoga Principles	1

    What are Yoga Principles?
    The Book is the Tool, You are the Guru

2	Chapter Two: Applying Yoga Principles to Stress and Anxiety	6

    Stress is your Friend, or it was before Modern Living
    How Stress affects your life, health and happiness
    Measuring what causes your stress
    Unhealthy Responses to Stress

3	Chapter Three: The Physical Plane – Your Body	13

    How does Your Body feel every day?
    The three Doshas: Vata, Pitta, and Kapha
    Vata Dosha
    Pitta Dosha
    Kapha Dosha
    Exercise: A way to reduce anxiety and release stress tension
    Hatha Yoga: Physical exercises to reduce stress
    Standing Downward bend or Uttanasana
    Downward facing Dog or Adho Mukha Svanasana
    Child's Pose or Baalasana
    Bridge pose or Setu bandha Sarvangasana
    Corpse Pose or Shavasana
    Belly Breathing: Your link between planes

4	**Chapter Four: The Physical Plane – Your Environment**	30

What do you see every day?
Vaastu, what your physical world does to your mental world
What is Vaastu?
What you can do to create a calm, peaceful environment using Vaastu
Your Entrance, the Gateway to your Home
Your bedroom, your Relaxation sanctuary

5	**Chapter Five: The Physical Plane – Your Rituals and Routines**	39

What do you do every day?
Rituals and Traditions
Rituals
Traditions
Routines
Creating your Sacred Space
Space clearing
Designing your Personal Yantra or Mandala

6	**Chapter Six: Your Meditation Practice**	52

An Introduction to Chakra Meditation
Why are these Chakras important?
Is it safe?
How do you do Chakra Meditation?
Your Chakras
The Chakras that might be affecting your Stress and Anxiety
Your Root Chakra
How to balance your Root Chakra
Walking meditation
Your Sacral Chakra
How to balance your Sacral Chakra
Flower Gazing

7   **Chapter Seven: The Emotional Plane – Battling Your Feelings**   65

    Emotions and Stress
    Apathy or the inability to feel
    Witnessing your emotions
    The Battle with Fear
    Gratitude
    Appreciation
    Desires and the Bhagwad Geeta

8   **Chapter Eight: The Mental Plane – Your Myths and Legends**   74

    Your thoughts create your world
    Your Problems
    Victimhood
    The Pollyana Syndrome
    New myths and legends
    Visualization
    Responsibility vs. Fate: The Bhagvad Geeta revisited

9   **Chapter Nine: Your Spiritual Plane – Your Consciousness and how You View the World**   86

    Experiencing the sacred in daily life
    As Above, So below
    Living with Integrity

ACKNOWLEDGMENTS

I would like to acknowledge my Guru who introduced me to these principles. My friends and family who spent hours reading, critiquing and editing my work and finally to my husband who has been a true support and a loving companion. Love, light and blessings to you all.

CHAPTER ONE: YOGA PRINCIPLES

What are Yoga Principles?

A long time ago in the subcontinent of India, a chosen few studied yoga to gain enlightenment. This yoga encompassed the five "types" of yoga that we know today. In ancient India, if you were a master of yoga you were a master of your body, mind and spirit.

Fast forward to today: Yoga has become a popular form of exercise. The most popular forms of yoga in the western world are all types of "hatha yoga" or yoga involving the body. The word "yoga" means to yolk or to join. Hatha Yoga is the union of the two major energy meridians or Nadi. Your left half of your body was called Ida or "tha" meaning moon. Your right half of your body was called Pingala or "ha".

Chapter One: Yoga Principles

Today, most people are aware only of the physical benefits yoga, but Bikram, Vinyasa or Iyengar are just different versions of Hatha or physical yoga. Many styles, such as Ashtanga, are based in Raja yoga and include meditation, chanting and breathing. But other styles of Yoga just see yoga as an exercise and a good way of maintaining your fitness.

Yoga is a systematic way of moving your body and mind towards more and more subtle forms of consciousness. These other levels are not a hierarchy but interact with each other.

There are four main systems that integrate to form your full self. These systems are Physical (also called Gross Body), Emotional, Mental (both make up the Subtle Body) and your subconscious and spirit which make up your Spiritual Body.

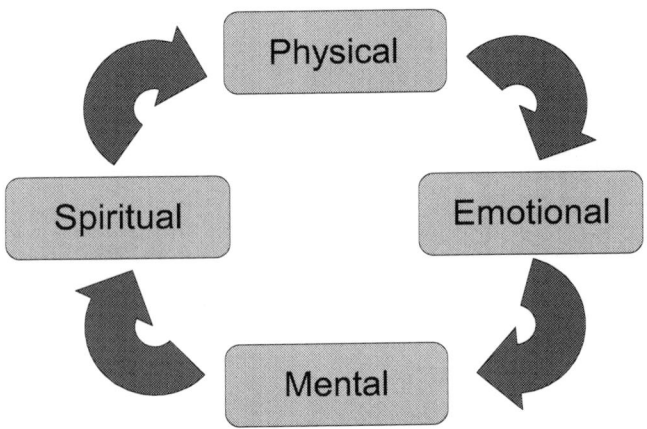

The Physical level: this includes your physical environment, your body and day-to-day activities

The Emotional level: this is your instinctual reactions to events and thoughts

The Mental level: this is where your ideas and thoughts originate

The Spiritual level: this is the seer, observer and your true self

When you start yoga, the physical level is only the beginning. You enter your emotional, mental and then spiritual level. So in traditional yoga, many years ago, yoga poses were a way of disciplining your body. Each pose had a mantra and specific breathing techniques to accompany it. As your body flowed from one pose to another you would train your brain with the various mantras then this made you aware of your emotions, and your thoughts. Controlling your thoughts then allowed you to experience "no thought" or as Buddhists say "no mind". And then, at this level you began to experience bliss and oneness with the universe. Of course this in turn can directly and immediately affect your body and your physical world.

The book is the tool, you are the Guru

In this book, we look at reducing your stress in the same way. The book begins by exploring your physical level. This includes yoga poses for you to practice to help you reduce stress, lifestyle changes that you may need to make, recommendations on what

Chapter One: Yoga Principles

you eat and arranging your environment to create sacred spaces through Vaastu. You will explore your habits in life to find your stressors. You will feel immediate relief from these activities but this book does not only reduce the symptoms. We will go deeper into the root of your anxiety and stress, your thoughts and emotions. Here you can create longer lasting changes to your stress and anxiety levels.

You will learn the emotional impact that anxiety and stress has on your life and what you can do to understand and even control your emotions.

Your mental plane comes next, and you will explore the triggers that cause your negative mental feedback and how to use your thoughts to help you reclaim your life in a positive way.

Finally, we will touch upon your spirit, what you can do to nurture it and how to use your spirit to support your physical practices.

Although this book uses Yoga and Indian philosophies, it also incorporates the body of research on stress and medically proven ways to reduce stress and anxiety.

This book does not have all the answers. You do. This book, accompanying workbook and guided meditations are only tools that you will use to manage your anxiety and stress. This means that you are the expert on what triggers your stress and what can work for you.

Your Peace Diet

I called this book *Your Peace Diet* because this book is just a "menu" of tools and insights that you can use in any combination that is best for you. The one catch? You must use these tools every day. If you do, then you will reduce your stress and less stress means a longer and happier life!

Okay, let's look at what stress is and how yoga principles can help stop it in its tracks.

CHAPTER TWO: APPLYING YOGA PRINCIPLES TO STRESS AND ANXIETY

If you're like me, you may not even remember that you're stressed, but I'm sure you feel the effects of it. Stress causes your muscles to start feeling sore, the tension in your neck and shoulders, stress causes you to have trouble sleeping or lose your temper easily. Maybe you have Irritable Bowel Syndrome or can't concentrate or remember things the way you used to. Yup, you guessed it. Another sign of stress. Fatigue is my sign that I'm stressed. So exactly what is stress? Why do we have stress and how do we get rid of it?

Stress is your friend, or it was before modern living

Stress is "pressure". When you put stress on an object you're applying pressure. This is also what happens with your body. Believe it or not, stress is our friend. It's one of our survival mechanisms. So getting rid of stress is close to impossible so don't feel bad if you're not in a constant state of Zen. But there are ways to manage and reduce stress.

Let's imagine we were a hunter or gatherer back thousands of years ago. You are going about your business when you hear some rustling in the woods. You freeze and your ears strain to listen. You body is on the alert. Ready for flight or fight. You pick up a rock ready to kill, but you stay alert just in case you couldn't kill it. The rustling gets louder and louder and out comes... your friend, Paul. You drop the rock and happily greet him. Your stress response disappears.

Now imagine you're in this time. You've got to walk the dog. The dog is bigger than you are and all of a sudden drags you out on the road. A car comes barreling round the corner honking the horn for you to get out of the way. You move. Fast. Miraculously pulling Fido out of harm's way. Stress allows your body to react faster to danger and without much thought.

Now what's the same about these situations? They're similar because there is a concrete or physical cause to the stress. Once you remove the stressor, your stress eventually returns to a normal level. This of course depends on how stressful the event was.

The problem with stress today is that stressors do not get resolved or removed.

Chapter Two: Applying Yoga Principles to Stress and Anxiety

The stress from your environment, your thoughts and emotions occur are mostly from **abstract** dangers such as not making enough money, losing your job, having your partner leave you or your friends hurt you. This then turns into a feedback loop which you play and replay like music in the back of your mind. Stress doesn't get removed like it does in concrete events. Instead, abstract stress constantly puts your body and mind under pressure.

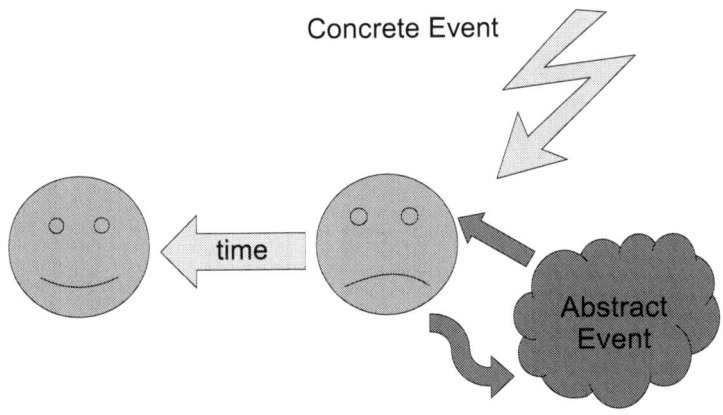

How stress affects your life, health and happiness

Here are some typical physical reactions to the fight and flight response:

- increased heart and breathing rate

- change in blood flow (constriction or dilation) in many parts of the body
- release of glucose into your muscles
- constriction of your saliva and tear ducts
- your bladder relaxes
- hearing loss
- tunnel vision
- quicker reflexes
- shaking
- release of adrenaline

The trouble is that our body needs a rest from these responses. Symptoms of chronic stress affect every part of your body. Being in this state can cause:

- depression
- irritable bowel syndrome
- heart palpitations
- shortness of breath
- feelings of being "weak" or tired

Chapter Two: Applying Yoga Principles to Stress and Anxiety

- nausea, abdominal pain and other digestive issues
- headaches
- insomnia
- depression
- gingivitis
- backaches
- intense mood swings
- loss of concentration
- increased confusion
- hypertension
- hemorrhoids
- suicidal thoughts

Are you experiencing any of these symptoms?

Measuring what causes your stress

The lists above tell you what typical symptoms are with the stress response as well as chronic stress. But you also need to find out what *your* stressors are. What causes *you* to experience these symptoms?

My stress level increases while I drive and in a crowded mall. I'm happy waiting in line which can drive other people crazy.

If you have the workbook, you can use the stress test to see what triggers a stress response in you. Otherwise, you need to collect data. First imagine yourself in common stressful situations and think back to if it caused any stress symptoms. If you are willing, you can put yourself in certain non-threatening situations or go through your day and observe what causes your stress response.

Stressors can be broken down into five main categories:

- Environmental (loud noises, bright lights, crowds)
- Daily stress events (waiting in traffic or in line, losing your keys or glasses)
- Workplace (deadlines, annoying co-workers)
- Life Changes (Divorce, Marriage, Baby, Bereavement)
- Bureaucratic stress (taxes, minor legal issues, etc.)

Unhealthy Responses to Stress

I congratulate you for seeing the value in forming healthy responses to stress. Many people are stressed or anxious and

Chapter Two: Applying Yoga Principles to Stress and Anxiety

instead choose unhealthy responses. Things like overeating, lack of exercise, binge drinking, smoking, consuming too much caffeine and overspending are pretty unhealthy ways of dealing with stress and anxiety and they lead to even more stress and anxiety. Let's see if we can find better alternatives shall we?

CHAPTER THREE: THE PHYSICAL PLANE - YOUR BODY

With chronic stress and anxiety, you can experience strong reactions in your body. Symptoms like not breathing properly, feeling weak, fatigued, suffering from headaches and backaches. Being in pain does not make you feel like taking care of your body. And exercise?? No way, out of the question.

First, use the workbook and find out if your body is suffering due to stress. Are you in pain? How are your eating and sleeping habits? Yes, it's a lot of writing down to do, but this way you can pinpoint what the effects of stress and anxiety are having on your body.

How does your body feel every day?

Is your body constantly aching? What about fatigue? Stress can cause chronic fatigue. Maybe you're feeling like this:

Chapter Three: The Physical Plane – Your Body

You work through your day, but feel tired for most of it. You wake up tired and go to bed exhausted, but you can't sleep.

Is this you? If it is, your body is out of balance.

What about this?

You're wired and alert; you love your caffeine and can't start the day without it. You're happiest when you're constantly on the go. Is this you? Unless you were born this way your body is also out of balance.

You should have enough energy for your whole day. Normally you feel a little dip after lunch time, but nothing you can't handle. By bed time you're tired and can fall asleep in under twenty minutes. Sleep refreshes you and makes you feel prepared for the next day.

Sounds like paradise? Well it should be the norm and if it isn't that means that something is not working right. So let's start off with learning more about your body, the yoga way.

The three Doshas: Vata, Pitta, and Kapha

Aryuveda is an ancient Indian form of diagnosing and preventing disease. In Aryuveda, your body is made up of the five elements.

Air/Space or **Vata**

Your Peace Diet

Fire/Water or **Pitta** and

Water/Earth, **Kapha**

Although all three doshas exist in your body, one of them will be dominant.

Find out what your dominant element is using the workbook. Oh and a small percent of the population is equally balanced in more than one Dosha. If you are, just go with the one that feels right for you.

Doshas are part of Aryuvedic medicine. Aryuveda means the study of long life and an Aryuvedic doctor studies your body and overall health in great detail. We will only be scratching the surface of this rich form of alternative medicine.

Now that you know your Dosha, I will explain what each Dosha is, what it looks like in balance and out of balance and gives general recommendations for each Dosha. If you are a combination or both, then you can choose which routine works best for you. This does not mean you shouldn't be seeking medical help. So don't miss any checkups or anything okay? Even though one of the Doshas is your dominant one, changes in your environment, seasons and other things affect your Doshas as well. So it's a good thing to read about all three Doshas.

Chapter Three: The Physical Plane – Your Body

Vata Dosha

Vata has the properties of air and space. When Vata is in balance, you are lively and charming, quick-witted and sharp. You may not sleep as much as others and you will need to eat small meals and often. You need to keep your body warm.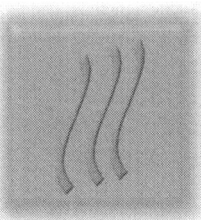

If your Vata Dosha is out of balance you will begin to feel anxious or worried. You cannot relax and you can't seem to fall asleep. Your skin and throat feel dry and you will have digestion problems. Are you experiencing any of these problems?

Let's look at ways you may be putting this Dosha out of balance.

- Have you recently been eating too much dry or raw food?

- Maybe consuming too many ice cold drinks?

- Have you been doing a lot of traveling recently?

- Or just had a major change in your lifestyle or routine?

Your Peace Diet

If any of these sound familiar, then you have an unbalanced Vata Dosha. Don't worry; balancing your Doshas is easy. Here are ways to balance your Vata Dosha:

Diet

Eat more warm, cooked food with a small amount of fat or oil in it. Soups are ideal for this; maybe try a cream of mushroom or chicken soup, yum! They're delicious, comforting and still good for you.

Sweet, sour or salty foods help balance Vata as well as spices. Here is a short list of foods that help balance Vata.

- Nuts
- Milk
- Citrus
- Basmati Rice
- Ghee
- Carrots
- Beets
- Potatoes, squash, zucchini
- Spinach

Chapter Three: The Physical Plane – Your Body

Other

You need a regular, daily routine. An out of balance Vata makes you feel like things are spinning out of control. For now, go to bed early to get as much sleep as you can.

Take extra care of your skin and use warmed oil to massage yourself after a warm shower or bath. Wear warm clothing and socks and a hat and scarf in cold weather.

Finally an early morning exercise routine which involves gentle exercise such as walking is best for Vata.

If you live in a seasonal environment, then Vata can get out of balance when the weather is changing such as in spring and autumn.

Pitta Dosha

Pitta has the properties of fire. When Pitta is in balance you are intelligent, determined and ambitious. You are very athletic and enjoy participating in competitive sports. You enjoy cooler environments and are regular sleepers.

When Pitta is out of balance you become angry and irritated, critical of others and argue a lot. You may also suffer from heartburn or skin irritations.

Here are ways you may be putting this Dosha out of balance.

Your Peace Diet

- Have you been eating too much hot, spicy food?
- Are you skipping meals?
- Have you recently been in a very hot environment?
- Have you just experienced some kind of emotional upset?
- Are you in an environment that makes you more irritable, critical or "hot under the collar" than usual?

All of this puts Pitta out of balance.

Diet

This diet is the opposite of Vata. You need to eat more dry and cooling food. Yoghurt is a good choice. Also sweet foods will help balance Pitta.

Sweet, bitter and cooling are the tastes that balance Pitta. Here are some foods that will help:

- Cucumber
- Avocado
- Pomegranate
- Yoghurt
- Dry cereal or crackers

Chapter Three: The Physical Plane – Your Body

- Broccoli
- Cauliflower
- Milk
- Drink lots of Cool (not cold) water

Other

The main thing with Pitta is to not overheat. Stay cool by not going out in very hot weather and wearing cotton or breathable clothing.

Eat regularly and do not skip meals. Skipping any meals can lead to heartburn, acid reflux or any symptoms of having high acidity in your stomach.

Use coconut oil to massage your body before you shower and do not take very hot showers.

Water sports or a late evening walk when it is cool helps balance Pitta.

Make sure that you take time out every day for play or non-goal oriented activities.

Your Pitta may be out of balance if you live in a very hot country or it's summer time in a seasonal country.

Kapha Dosha

Although my body is balanced between the three Doshas, I am "spiritually" Kapha Dosha. Kapha Dosha is a combination of Water and Earth (and yes, if you combine them you get mud).

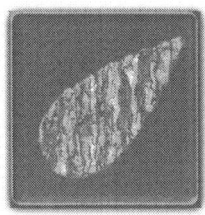

If you are a Kapha Dosha in balance, you are easygoing, loving and slow to anger. You are stable and serene and enjoy warm, dry environments. And boy do you love your sleep!

If Kapha is out of balance, you feel sluggish and slow and being a bit "stuck in the mud". You feel a bit lazy and just want to withdraw from the world.

Here are some ways you'd put Kapha out of balance:

- Have you been eating too many oily, deep-fried or sweet foods?
- Have you been doing the "same old routine" for too long?
- Have you been feeling depressed?
- Have you stopped exercising recently?
- Has the weather recently been rainy or very damp?
- Are you congested in your throat, nose or chest?

Chapter Three: The Physical Plane – Your Body

All of this means that Kapha is out of balance.

Diet

If Kapha is out of balance you need to eat dry, warm food. Dhal or bean soups are good for this; just add fresh herbs and spices instead of salt. Also avoid oily or sweet foods.

Pungent, bitter and astringent are the tastes that balance Kapha. Here are some foods that will help:

- buckwheat
- quinoa
- asparagus
- lemons and limes
- fresh herbs and herbal tea
- Mung beans and chickpeas
- Use only a little honey, no other sweetener
- ginger
- turmeric

Other

Vigorous exercise is the best thing to do for this Dosha, if that seems like too much at least brisk walking for 20-30 minutes every morning will help.

Vary your routine and take up a stimulating mental or physical hobby such as martial arts, yoga, painting, drawing or writing.

Meeting new people may sound daunting but becoming a volunteer is perfect for the nurturing Kapha.

Exfoliating your skin by using a granulated cream before your morning shower will help you feel more alive and gets you out of your rut.

Try not to nap in the daytime, at least until you are able to easily fall asleep at night and wake up easily in the morning.

Exercise: A way to reduce anxiety and release stress tension

I know for some of you this is the last thing you feel like doing when you're stressed or anxious, but I cannot emphasize enough how important exercise is for you especially at this time. Here are a few reasons that you should think of exercising even if you don't feel like it.

- Regulates your heart so you don't experience heart palpitations.

Chapter Three: The Physical Plane – Your Body

- Fatigues your muscles so your muscles don't tense up. This can relieve stress tension.

- Increases your metabolism

- Regulates your serotonin and melatonin so you feel tired

- Strengthens your bones

Exercising does not always have to be vigorous. You should make it fun time. If you are interested go to a yoga, Zumba®, a dance class or try a sport that you might enjoy like tennis, golf, martial arts or running. Exercise does not mean that you have to be in a gym, sweating away, going nowhere on the treadmill.

Hatha Yoga: Physical exercises to reduce stress

Here are some yoga asanas or poses which can help with stress and anxiety:

Most inverted or restorative poses will help. Here is a short sequence of five yoga poses that can help you reduce stress. Remember to do this on an empty stomach. So either before a meal or 2-3 hours after eating.

Your Peace Diet

Standing Downward bend or Uttanasana

Stand tall.

Raise your arms straight over your head, straighten your spine as much as you can and feel like you're touching the sky.

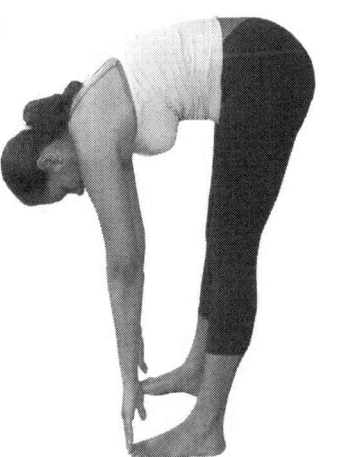

Bend from your hip sockets gently down as far as you can go.

Bend your knees. **The object of this pose is not to see if you can touch the floor or put your head between your knees, but to get a nice stretch in the back of the legs and spine.** Five belly breaths in this posture.

If this is still too difficult then it is better to do a sitting forward bend. Sit and do this pose. Keep your feet flexed. Remember, just get a nice stretch.

Downward facing Dog or Adho Mukha Svanasana

In Forward bend, bend your knees and walk your hands out to where it is comfortable. Your hands should feel firmly planted on the floor. Your feet should be shoulder width apart. Lift your hips up and pull your shoulder blades up toward your waist.

Chapter Three: The Physical Plane – Your Body

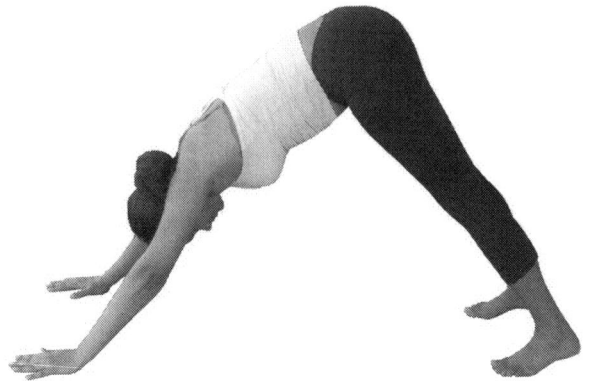

This pose should stretch out your back and arms and keep your arms straight. If you can (I can't!) straighten your legs and put your heels on the floor.

Work up to five breaths in this posture.

Child's Pose or Baalasana

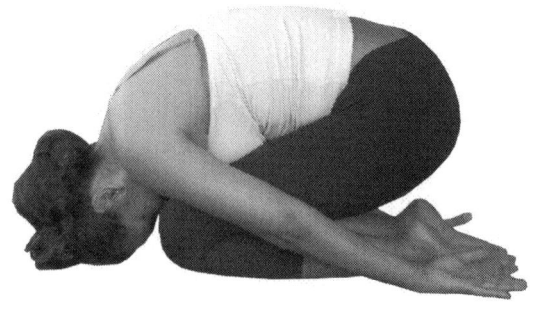

This pose is great for stretching your back and relaxing your body. Don't do this on a full stomach as this pose puts pressure on your abs.

Start with downward facing dog. On an exhale, bend your knees until you are sitting on your calves.

Put your head to the floor if you can and hands to your sides, palm up. Stay for three to five breaths.

Bridge pose or Setu bandha Sarvangasana

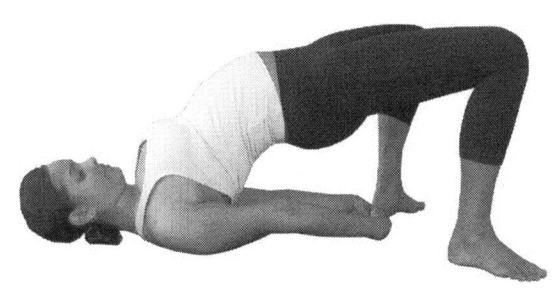

Lie down on your back with your knees bent. Press your feet on the floor and lift your pelvis. Now roll your shoulder blades in towards the floor.

Join your hands together and push downwards. Breathe in and lift your chest. Hold for two to five breaths.

Corpse Pose or Shavasana

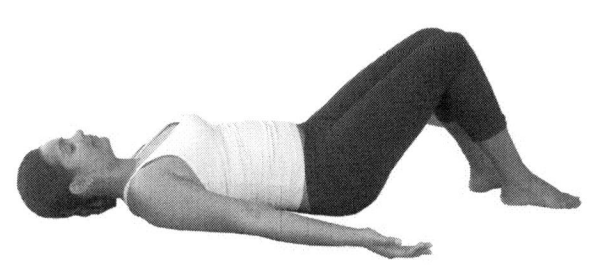

This is a restorative pose. It's called "corpse" or dead man's pose because all the parts of your body is at rest and neutral.

Chapter Three: The Physical Plane – Your Body

First lie on your back. If you have back pain, bend your knees. Breathe deeply from your abdomen. Stay in this pose for 3-5 minutes.

Other poses you may like to try:

- **Shoulder stand Pose**
- **Plough Pose**
- **Cobra Pose**
- **Supported Headstand**

Belly Breathing: Your link between planes

Do you suffer from anxiety attacks? Does your heart race and your pulse quicken often? Do you get stressed easily? Belly breathing is a quick way to stop and slow down. It has an almost immediate effect on your body and if you concentrate on your breathing, it can calm your mind as well.

Of course, you must know how to do belly breaths properly. Make sure you practice it regularly so that it becomes second nature and you can use it in stressful situations.

Let your abdomen relax. When you breathe in, try not to move your shoulders and chest, but have your belly or abs do the work. Feel your diaphragm (which is located under the lungs) lower as your lungs fill with air. On your exhale, feel your ribs draw together. Relax your stomach again and repeat two more times, observing the flow of air.

If you can't get the air to flow down to your abdomen, imagine the air flowing down your spine to as low as you feel comfortable. Just don't let your chest rise.

Practice belly breaths regularly. In the car at the traffic light, when you're on the computer or any time you have a free minute. Remember to relax your abs.

Remember to keep practicing; this is the best thing to do during moments of stress or anxiety. It stops the "deadly" spiral of worry in its tracks.

Next let's look at your environment and if it is affecting your stress and anxiety.

CHAPTER FOUR: THE PHYSICAL PLANE - YOUR ENVIRONMENT

Do you spend all morning trying to find your keys? Maybe you need to dress up for a special occasion and when you look through your overstuffed wardrobe; you realize that you have nothing to wear. Are there parts of your home or entire rooms where you just want to close the door because of all the clutter?

Sounds familiar? If so, your environment is holding you back from living the peaceful, joyful life that you deserve. Don't believe that an orderly room can have an effect on your emotions? Have you ever walked around a

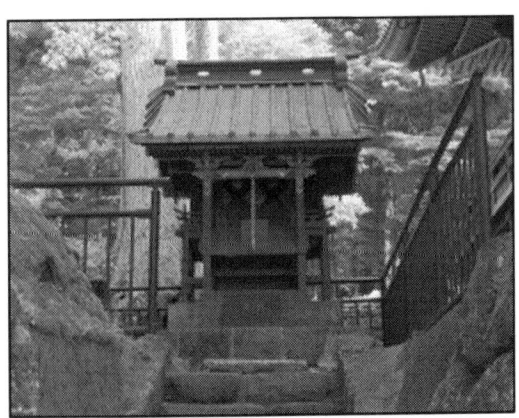

Zen garden? Part of what makes it so peaceful is the attention to detail and the extreme attention to detail, the orderliness of the items.

Maybe your house is in order but you feel like things just aren't getting done. Are there too many little things to do? Do you feel overwhelmed? This is also part of your environment but we'll talk about that in another chapter.

What do you see every day?

What you see every day contributes to your stress and if things don't "feel" restful and harmonious when you look around, it increases your stress response.

How does your environment affect your stress levels? Chronic stress is a result of small things that annoy you every day and not being able to find things and have easy access to rooms, storage etc. Whatever it is that gives you that nagging feeling is worse for your health than a big concrete stressor. These small chronic stresses can take years off your life.

This part of the book looks at which parts of your home may cause your stress and how to infuse your home and environment with things (or lack of things) that brings you a sense of calm and contentment. You don't have to redecorate or redo your entire house. Just start with one space, your sacred space. You will fill that space with beauty, serenity and it will allow you to fully relax your body and your mind.

Chapter Four: The Physical Plane – Your Environment

Vaastu, what your physical world does to your mental world

What is Vaastu?

Vaastu is the ancient science of space and architecture. If you lived in India hundreds of years ago and you were fairly wealthy, you would consult a Vaastu practitioner before building your home and to survey your plot of land. Most Indian temples still use Vaastu before the ground is even broken.

Vaastu believes that the reason there is life on this planet is because there is a balance of the five elements. These elements are:

- **Earth** (Bhumi) furniture, "weight" of room
- **Water** (Jal) Coolness, darkness, yin energy
- **Fire** (Agni) light and heat, yang energy
- **Air** (Vaayu) circulation
- **Space** (Aakaash) space to live, amount of clutter

Kind of looks familiar doesn't it? Doshas and Chakras are also related to these five elements.

The trick is to keep these five elements balanced. If you have all five elements in harmony, your home, building or temple will also be harmonious. If these five elements are balanced and

Your Peace Diet

your home is clutter free, Prana (similar to Chi in Feng Shui) can then circulate freely and promote joy, prosperity and harmony.

Vaastu also looks at the cardinal directions which are governed by various "gods". Examples of these are:

- The **North** is ruled by Kubera – deity of wealth
- The **South** is ruled by Yama – deity of death
- The **East** is ruled by Indra and Aditya – deities of the sun and vision
- The **West** is ruled by Varuna – the deity of water
- The **Northeast** is ruled by Shiva (a good place for meditation and spiritual pursuits)
- The **Southeast** is ruled by Agni – the deity of fire
- The **Northwest** is ruled by Vayu – the deity of wind or air
- The **Southwest** is ruled by Pitri/Niruthi – or your ancestors
- The **Center** of the home is ruled by Brahma – the creator of the universe

Chapter Four: The Physical Plane – Your Environment

Vaastu has similarities and differences with Feng Shui. Many of the differences are to do with the environment of their country of origin.

For example, Feng Shui had to deal with cold winds coming from the North, whereas Vaastu had to deal with the heat of the Indian climates. So a northern hill is favorable in Feng Shui and a disaster in Vaastu.

The principles of Vaastu and Feng Shui are similar in other ways. An example of this is that both state how you arrange your space will affect how much enjoyment you get in your home. Vaastu, like Aryuveda, is a science and we are just looking at a piece of it.

Don't worry though; I am not going to ask you to move your front door so it is facing east or any major renovations. In this chapter we will just look at some ideas to make your home a place of peace and relaxation.

What you can do to create a calm, peaceful environment using Vaastu

We will look at your home's entrance as well as your bedroom as examples, but you can apply this to your entire home if you wish. We will also look at balancing the five elements in your rooms.

Let's look at your physical environment. I would like you to note which areas of your environment give you the most stress.

Your Peace Diet

You can do this now with your workbook. Visit each room. What is the main function of this room? Is it fulfilling that function? How easy is it to move around your room? Is your room balanced? Does it have a place for everything?

Now I am not a neat person. I don't believe that you need to have a sterile or bare environment to find peace, but if you spend two minutes looking for your keys in the morning that adds up to over 12 hours a year!

Take note of the rooms that cause you the most stress. Do items need to be fixed? Are things in major disarray? (It is major disarray if you look for more than three minutes for an item on most days). Take note of what needs to be done. Keep in mind that this nagging clutter is taking years off your life! Use the workbook and action plan to get this complete.

Your Entrance, the Gateway to your Home

Now I want you to look at the **entrance** to your home. Think of these things specifically. Where can I put items that I need when I am entering or leaving the house? Do I have enough room for everything that is there?

The reason that we focus on your entrance is that the entrance to you home sets your emotional tone or mood when you enter and you want it filled with peace and joy, not stress. Put something there that will make you smile. Have a place to put your keys, maybe fresh flowers, or beautiful artwork and keep

Chapter Four: The Physical Plane – Your Environment

shoes, jackets etc. in a closet or neatly stacked out of the way. I would also recommend having a paper recycle bin for those unwanted mail ads.

Your bedroom, your Relaxation sanctuary

Now according to traditional Vaastu there are things that you need to arrange in your bedroom to have a good night's sleep.

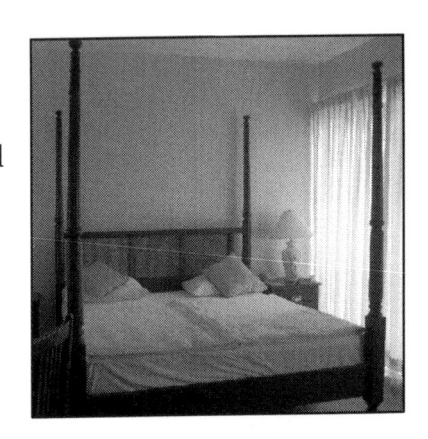

Here are a few:

- Sleep with your head towards the South or East side (I was taught as a little girl that your feet face South only for your funeral! Yikes!)
- Do not sleep under exposed beams (same as Feng Shui)
- Keep electronics or gadgets to a minimum and keep it away from the bed.
- Do not keep iron or metal under your bed
- Cover all exposed mirrors and screens
- Keep the bed three feet away from the wall.

Does it sound a bit random? There are practical reasons for some of these ideas. For example, keeping the room as electronics free as possible. This is because most electronics today emit some form of blue light. This blue light is terrible for sleep.

Why? Because studies show that light, especially blue light, increases your cortisol levels, decreases your melatonin levels and can interrupt your sleep. So those blue computer lights from your shiny new iPad might be doing a number on your sleep patterns.

This is also why you should try not to watch television or use the computer when in bed. Also, when you sleep, keep the room as dark as possible. I am guessing that covering the mirrors is also a way to keep the room dark.

Do you enjoy sleeping in your bedroom? Is your bed comfortable? Are you using the right pillow for your sleeping style? And is your room clutter (not personality) free? Try to open the windows of your bedroom during the day as often as you can to allow air to circulate. I know that it is more difficult for you if you live in a country with a terrible winter, but even 10 minutes will help.

Here are the five elements to use as a checklist:

Earth: Does your bed feel solid and grounded?

Water: Can the room be dark at night? Is it painted in a calm color?

Fire: Does it get enough natural light during the day?

Air: Is your bedroom too stuffy?

Chapter Four: The Physical Plane – Your Environment

Space: Can you move freely from your bed to other parts of the room? To other parts of the house?

Hopefully, you can take these examples and use them throughout your house. Remember, clutter holds energy (Prana or Chi) and energy should circulate throughout your home instead of getting stuck.

Next, let's move on to some of the routines that you have in your everyday life that may be aggravating your stress levels.

CHAPTER FIVE: THE PHYSICAL PLANE – YOUR RITUALS AND ROUTINES

Rituals sound like I'm going to take you to a pagan ceremony doesn't it? It conjures up images of people in long robes and masks. But the rituals that I am referring to are just a regular set of actions that have symbolic value behind them.

For example, my husband loves coffee. If he could grow viable coffee beans, he would. He buys green coffee beans and roasts them to his preference, grinds them just before he makes the coffee and then uses a machine that costs thousands of dollars to create his perfect cup. Even I admit, he makes excellent coffee.

Is this a ritual? Absolutely. Why? Because it isn't about the coffee alone. It symbolizes a break in routine, a physical mindless set of actions that brings my husband pleasure, a break from his computer work and something delicious to have.

Chapter Five: The Physical Plane – Your Rituals and Routines

Can rituals be bad for you? Yes. Can they be healthy and wonderful? Also Yes. We will be exploring your rituals to see if you have any that are stressing you out and what you can do to develop positive, peaceful rituals.

The other things that we will look at in this chapter are your routines. Again, you may think that I'm going to prescribe a set of routines or a schedule that I think that you need to start today to have a happy, healthy life. But I'm a firm believer in "everyone is as unique as their fingerprint". You need to look at the routines in your life that aren't serving you and develop ones that work best for you and your life now. You can change them as your life continues to grow and develop (and you are always growing and developing).

What do you do every day?

First I would like you to take a look at what you do every day. Keep a look out for things that are rituals (such as eating for comfort not for energy) and routines like what you do to get yourself out the door in the morning or what you do when you get home after a hard day's work. I want you to base if what you are doing is worth it on one thing only.

Is it making you happy?

How do you know? Well like true scientists we are going to observe your life for a week and find out. I call it the *Happiness Analysis*. It is a lot of work. I want you to take twenty minutes out of your day (five minutes x four times), look at what you're doing and rate it on a Happiness Scale. I want you to do this for a week. Why? Because there are such things as the Monday blues, sick children, a getaway weekend and lots of things that can throw this off. But if you do it for seven days, you will truly find out what really makes you happy. What you find out may surprise you.

Are you willing to do the work to remove the stress in your life for good? Look for the *Happiness Analysis* in the workbook and then analyze the results.

Now you have a starting point to build new rituals and routines and remove old ones that are not serving your needs.

Rituals and Traditions

Now that you know a little more about rituals and routines as well as areas of your life where you can start creating better rituals and routines. Let's take a look at ways that you can begin to create rituals and routines that serve you.

Rituals

First, do you have a daily ritual? Something that signals that you are finished working and ready to relax or play? Or are the lines blurred?

Let's use the idea of having a daily ritual to signal that you are finished with work. Mentally, physically and emotionally and

Chapter Five: The Physical Plane – Your Rituals and Routines

are ready to be present at home, with your family, friends and children.

If you work from home like me, or if you are in a profession where you take work home (and that means mentally as well as physically) your lines between work time and play time are blurred. You need a ritual to signal to yourself that you are finished with work and ready to play. Similarly, in the morning you need a ritual to get you into work-ready mode. Let's start with beginning work. How do you start work? Do you open up your computer and look at your emails? (I tend to do that, it is not a positive ritual, but it does signal work for me). Do you have a meeting? A to-do or action list? Or do you just dive into work?

The healthiest ritual to begin work would be:

If you are an employee, coming into work in a happy relaxed manner and checking the action plan that you planned yesterday to see if anything needs updating.

For someone who runs a business, is self-employed or works from home the best thing to do is to review your action plan from yesterday and do the most pressing item on your list.

This involves one thing – taking time to plan your day. Planning is one of the rituals that I highly recommend to signal the close of the workday.

Your Peace Diet

Now when you get home, after negotiating your way through traffic, rushing to pick your children up from child care or especially if your commute is from one room to the other, you need to close the stresses of the day and begin relaxing even for a few minutes before starting your duties at home.

- Your rituals may include:
- Having a cool or hot drink
- Changing your clothes
- Sitting and looking through your mail
- Meditating
- Sitting and chatting with others about their day

Remember, just taking ten minutes to do this will help you to transition from work to home mode. The key is to recognize this transition. It doesn't have to be relaxing (but I enjoy it when it is!) but it has to clearly draw the line between work and home.

Take a few minutes to decide what your ritual will be. Write it down in your workbook.

Traditions

Traditions are different from rituals, though they may include rituals. An example is Christmas. Christmas is a famous series

Chapter Five: The Physical Plane – Your Rituals and Routines

of traditions even if you are not Christian. Countries all over the world take part in this holiday. Christmas trees, family gatherings and various versions of Santa Claus or Saint Nicholas abound in December.

Even though there are common threads, when I moved to New Zealand from Canada, wow, were some of the traditions different. No one had even heard of egg nog! And a barbeque is the most common Christmas dinner. I am surprised by how much Christmas in New Zealand doesn't "feel like Christmas" to me. The summer weather is a major part of it, but the traditions here are not the ones I grew up with.

So why am I talking about Christmas when you want to relieve stress and anxiety? "The Holidays" as it's called now is probably one of the most stressful times of the year. No, I don't intend to make you hyperventilate.

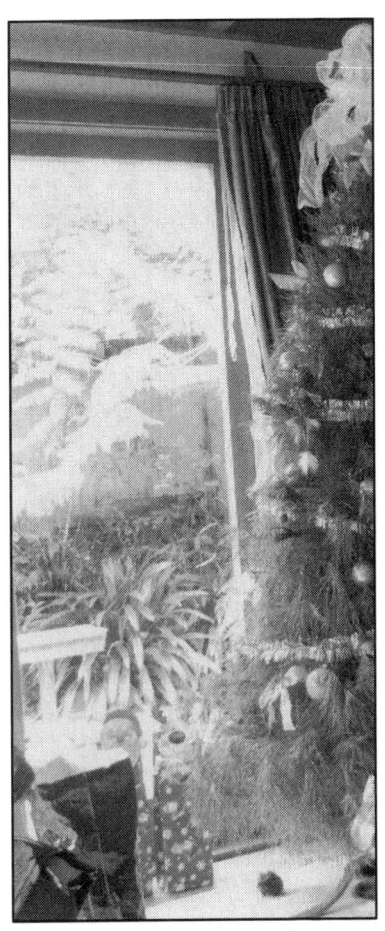

Your Peace Diet

I would instead, like to invite you to create Peace Traditions and build them into your life. The thing with traditions is that it had to start somewhere. Be creative and fun with starting this tradition. Maybe you can make it a weekly tradition to have a quiet hour (my parents successfully did this with three children). Hmm, not much fun? Maybe decide to have a monthly laughing party or a joke telling fest. Whatever you decide that reduces your stress and allows you to have fun with your family and friends. I'm sure you can be much more creative with this than I can.

Routines

Ah, another boring sounding word. Again it's something we do every day. What does your "getting ready for the morning" routine look like? Do you have enough time to relax in the morning? And no I'm not going to be encouraging you to get up an hour earlier to relax. Unless that's a goal that you want, I'm not going to force that extra worry on you. I'm just going to ask you one question. Is there anything you're doing in the morning that you could move to your "before bed" routine?

I found that even though I was tired, I still had time to do more things in the evening than in the morning. I even went as far as showering before bed as that gave me ten more minutes to relax in the morning. The idea of course is to still get up at the same time and not think that you have ten minutes more to sleep in. Just look through the routines that you have for stress "hot

Chapter Five: The Physical Plane – Your Rituals and Routines

spots". Being stressed first thing in the morning will set the tone for the rest of the day.

Also create routines that will stop stress. This sounds a bit embarrassing, but sing along to your favorite music on the way to work. The traffic will go by much more quickly.
Commuting? I used to love to catch up on my reading. Read something inspiring so you go into work excited. Do whatever it takes to make your mornings as stress free as possible.

Now let's look at some positive rituals that you can use to create more peace and less stress in your life.

Creating your Sacred Space

Most ancient religions have you create a space in your home. A space that encourages you to be the best you can be in that space. Many of these religions also have rituals that allow you to create a sacred space.

This space is very important in your life. You can enter this space and feel peace, connectedness and oneness with the world. It does not have to be a large space but must have some important elements:

- It must be clean and free of clutter
- It must be an inviting place to sit and stay for a while
- It should always be the same space

Your Peace Diet

- It must have objects that inspire you

This would be the place that you go to for meditation, when you feel anxious, worried or burdened with stress. It won't be a place for comfort however, unless you fill the space with a peaceful atmosphere.

You can use a corner of a room or an entire room, but it must be a space that has all those requirements. I personally like a space where:

- There aren't many distractions
- There is a view of nature or natural objects
- It has lots of natural light

Now that may not be what's best for you. You may prefer a place that is outdoors, a Zen garden or a dark room. You can add things that have strong personal meaning for you, things that make you happy or proud. A picture, your medals from third grade, anything. This space becomes sacred because it is personal to you. This is where you will go to meditate and practice yoga. Sit in this space every day with positive intentions so it becomes a positive environment, a place of solace to turn to when you need calm and peace.

Chapter Five: The Physical Plane – Your Rituals and Routines

Space clearing

Space clearing is a tradition where you clear the space of negative energy and encourage a positive energy flow. Both Asian and South Asian traditions have some form of this ritual when they buy a new home or occupy a new space. A space clearing is usually done when you move into a new home. However, you can do a space clearing whenever you need it. Here's what you'll need:

- Something to symbolize **Earth**: A clay pot, salt, or flowers will do.

- **Water** of any kind

- A candle or lamp to symbolizes **Fire**

- Bells, a gong or just a metal pot cover and a spoon as long as it makes a pleasant sound, this symbolizes **Air**

- Incense or something that smells nice and a good clean, room or rooms with symbolizes **Space**

Notice that this also indirectly involves your five senses. So of course you'd clean up the room or rooms that you would like to clear. Enjoy doing this. Think about the outcome that you want and have it clear in your mind. Imagine peaceful times,

Your Peace Diet

joy and lots of laughter. Keep this intention in mind when doing the rest of this ritual.

1. Then take the element of earth and if it is the salt or flowers, scatter it around the room. If it is the pot carry it around the room and set it down somewhere safe.

2. Next, sprinkle water around the room and set the container down in a safe place (sometimes I use a clay pot with water in it, two elements at once!).

3. Light the candle, hold it carefully and move it around the room, think of it as removing the darkness that may be there. Again place it in a safe surface. Do not leave the candle unattended.

4. Ring the bells and move the incense along in the same way.

5. Now imagine your best outcome for this room. Fill your mind full of happy thoughts.

6. Then you can put out the candle but leave everything in place for 24 hours before cleaning it up. This is where the elements absorb negative energy.

7. If you would like to say or chant things, it's up to you. I find holding a positive mental and emotional intention usually works best.

Designing your Personal Yantra or Mandala

Yantra means an instrument of restraint. It is used to describe a visual symbol made up of geometrical shapes. The Buddhist term for these series of shapes is Mandala or "circle". A mandala usually has a circle with a series of shapes that lead your eye into the center of the circle. This lets you to focus inward, so Yantra watching is a form of meditation. Focusing on a Yantra helps you to focus your mind on your emotions and spirituality. Each shape in a Yantra or Mandala has a symbolic meaning.

For example:

- Lotus flower= Chakras
- Dot = creation or beginnings
- Six pointed star or (shatkona)= balance between the masculine and the feminine, Yin and Yang
- Circle, horizontal lines = Water element
- Square, vertical lines = Earth element
- Triangle = Fire element
- Diagonal lines = Air element

Your Peace Diet

- Points = Space element

If you choose to create this symbol, you can apply the symbolism that I've given you or create your own. Think of this Yantra as a personal symbol and make sure to look at it every day to remind you of who you are and what you are capable of.

CHAPTER SIX: YOUR MEDITATION PRACTICE

Meditation begins to involve both your body and your mind. As we begin to cross from the physical plane into the mental, emotional and spiritual plane, I would like to introduce Chakra Meditation. This form of meditation is an excellent way to gauge your body's energy. After that, we'll discuss the Chakras that may be closed for you when you experience stress and anxiety and what you can do to focus on opening them.

An introduction to Chakra Meditation

Chakra meditation is a type of focused meditation. This style of meditation is used in Kundalini yoga, Tantra and Tibetan Buddhism. In this style of meditation you focus on points in your body called the Chakras.

These Chakras correspond with important organs and bundles of nerves or plexuses in your body. Chakra comes from the

Sanskrit word "wheel". This makes sense as a Chakra point is considered to be a swirling, moving wheel of energy.

Chakras are part of an ancient system which accepts that we have a physical or "gross" body and an energy or "subtle" body. The Chakras correspond to your energy body.

There are many different systems of Chakras. All of these systems have a few things in common.

- Chakras are energy centers

- The main Chakras are found along an energy line (Nadi) which corresponds to your spine

- Some systems like the Tibetan Vajrayana believe that each of the main Chakras break into points or spokes which branch out into thousands of Nadis or energy lines

- Chakras are associated with a mantra, symbol, color and deity

Why are these Chakras important?

There are two things that Chakras are used for. The first is that your Chakras are the means for your life force, chi or prana to increase its flow.

The second use is to open all of your Chakras and remove the granthas or knots that close the flow of energy upwards. In

Chapter Six: Your Meditation Practice

Kundalini yoga you open your energy centers from your Root Chakra to your crown Chakra to allow Kundalini to pass through. As each chakra become opened and balanced, Kundalini, which is represented by a serpent, awakens and flows through your body, uniting with God, or the universal energy. When this happens you become spiritually enlightened.

In Western theory your Chakras need to be opened and balanced – not over-stimulated or closed.

For example, if your Chakra is closed, say in your throat, you will not communicate well with others, and won't be able to speak "your truth". If your Chakra is over-stimulated you will dominate conversations and be prone to gossip.

Is it safe?

Chakras are very interesting. I am naturally inquisitive and although I'm not a skeptic, my husband is so I experience a nice balance. If I concentrate on the areas in my body where the Chakras are I do feel as if "energy" has opened up in that area. So there seems to be "something" going on. And it doesn't feel bad, it feels good.

So where's the problem?

Sometimes opening "energy centers" and having a surge of energy that your body can't handle causes what may feel like a psychotic episode or bad drug "trip". At least, this is what some people report when doing Kundalini yoga.

You also could over-stimulate your Chakra and put it out of balance.

I don't think that you should worry too much as a new chakra meditator as long as you don't push yourself. Meditation is just about letting things be, and most of these energy surges are from people pushing hard for that energy surge before their bodies are ready.

How do you do Chakra Meditation?

This is the method that was taught to me. First, start with your root Chakra, and picture the color, sound and what it represents. Visualize the light growing and swirling in a clockwise motion and once it feels opened and good, move on to the next Chakra.

All of your Chakras may open or some may remain closed. You'll need to be patient and gentle. Do not feel frustrated or push.

I would recommend doing Chakra meditation if you feel tired and need energy.

A focused Chakra meditation can help if one or more of your Chakras are closed. By picturing the corresponding colors and energy points in your body again very gently you may be able to open them. You can also close or balance your Chakras by imagining a dimming light and imagining the swirl of energy slow down.

Chapter Six: Your Meditation Practice

Your Chakras

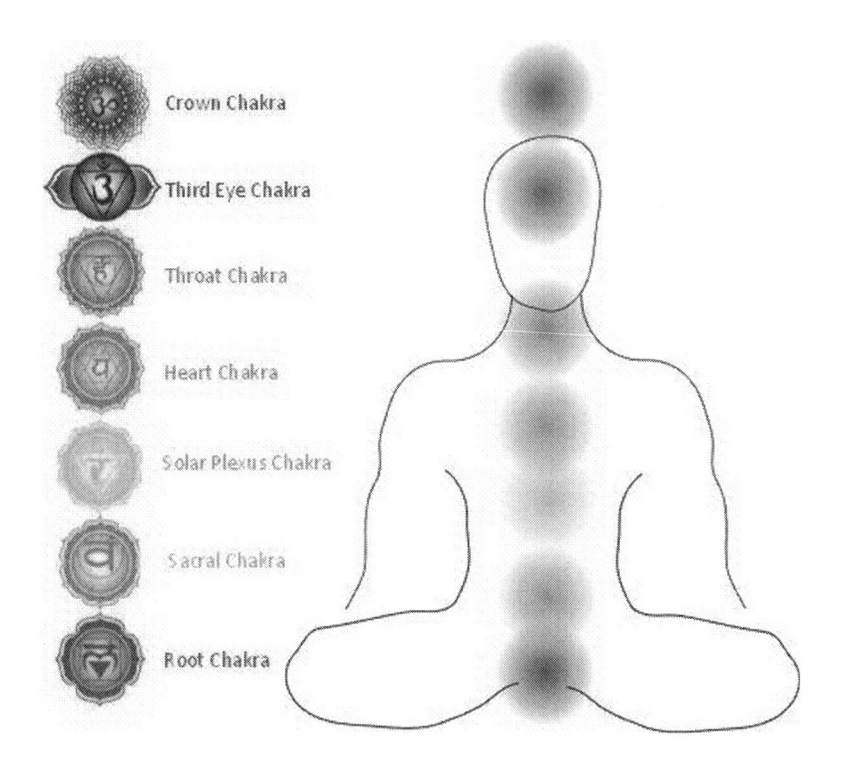

- Crown Chakra
- Third Eye Chakra
- Throat Chakra
- Heart Chakra
- Solar Plexus Chakra
- Sacral Chakra
- Root Chakra

As you can see in the Chakra chart, there are seven main Chakras along the main Nadi. These are:

The Root Chakra (Mulaadhaar)

This Chakra is located at the base of your spine. It is associated with security, instinct and survival. It is represented by the color red.

The Sacral Chakra (Swaadhisthhaan)

Located at the sacrum, this Chakra is associated with sexuality, relationships, addictions, basic needs and pleasure. I was told that this is your physical powerhouse and your joy and passion point. Its color is orange.

The Solar Plexus Chakra (Manipur)

This Chakra is found near the digestive system and solar plexus. This Chakra is your personal power center. This is where your belief in yourself, personal power, more complex emotions and self-confidence. The color associated with this Chakra is yellow.

The Heart Chakra (Anaahat)

Anahat yoga focuses solely on opening this Chakra. This Chakra is associated with your heart and all matters of love, caring for others and compassion. The color for this Chakra is green or pink.

The Throat Chakra (Vishuddh)

This Chakra is associated with your thyroid gland and helps you with being able to express yourself and communicate with others. Blue is the color that represents this Chakra.

Chapter Six: Your Meditation Practice

The Third Eye or Brow Chakra (Aangyaa)

This is the pineal gland Chakra and is associated with intuition. It helps balance your sleeping patterns and if you believe in psychic abilities, this Chakra is the one to help with that. Indigo is the color for this Chakra.

The Crown Chakra (Sahasraar)

This is associated with your brain and it is sometimes placed above your head, floating like a crown. This Chakra is about being visionary; it represents spiritual enlightenment and higher intelligence. It can be represented by gold, silver or white colors.

The Chakras that might be affecting your Stress and Anxiety

Now that you have been introduced to Chakras, and the Chakra system, we will focus on the Chakras that are most likely out of balance for you.

If you are feeling stressed or anxious, you're not feeling secure and grounded, you're probably not feeling joyful and you're not in your personal power. The Chakras that you need to focus on are the first two Chakras. Let's explore ways to balance and open these Chakras. If these Chakras are not open and balanced then working on other Chakras will be pointless.

Your Root Chakra

Your Root Chakra is called Mulaadhaar. It is located at the base of the spine. If you are sitting crossed-legged on the floor, this is the part of your back that touches the ground. This Chakra is associated with the earth element.

Many people when they first become interested in Chakras try to open their "third eye" Chakra or their "heart" Chakra first. They seem to pay very little attention to their root Chakra. This is a mistake. This Chakra grounds you. It keeps you level-headed and aware of the physical world around you. Remember, yoga is about balance. It is about uniting your spirituality and the physicality of living in this world. Your root Chakra also makes you feel secure. Feeling insecure causes you to feel anxious, worried and fearful. You cannot enjoy life without the feeling of being grounded and secure in this world.

How to balance your Root Chakra

I will make a few suggestions to open and balance your root Chakra; these are just guidelines and if you have other rituals to connect you with the physical world add it to the list. The intention of these exercises is to make you aware of the present moment and keep you present in life.

- Belly Breaths: doing this type of breathing makes you slow down and makes you more aware of your body.

Chapter Six: Your Meditation Practice

- Connecting with the earth. In the morning before climbing out of bed, be grateful for the earth and the ground that you walk on. Feel that the soles of your feet are sending and receiving energy from deep inside the earth. I was told as a girl that before I stepped on the ground I should thank mother earth (Dharti Maataa) for allowing me to walk on her body.

- Cleaning and reducing clutter in your home

- Walking barefoot (do it at least 15-20 minutes a day) this is very good for your feet and reducing things like corns, bunions and athlete's foot.

- Exercising

- Gardening

- Cooking

- If you believe in affirmations words such as "I have everything I need", "Life is good" or "I have a right to be here" are useful

Some of these suggestions should look familiar from earlier parts of the book.

Your Peace Diet

Walking meditation

A walking meditation will allow you to connect with both your body and the earth. Here are seven steps to a successful walking meditation:

Step 1: Make sure you are not in a hurry. Give yourself 20 minutes to finish the exercise

Step 2: Give yourself enough room to walk for 20 minutes where you will not be disturbed. Preferably on nice, flat terrain. An indoor walking track, an easy forest walk or a park with a path would be best.

Step 3: First stand tall, breathe in and on the out breath take a step. Try to be aware of the muscle movements in your body. Place your hands on your ab muscles during your first steps and then out to your sides or clasp your hands in front of you like a Buddhist Monk.

Step 4: Breathe, and focus on the flow of your breath.

Step 5: Do not try to exert yourself. You're not trying to exercise.

Step 6: Do not set yourself a goal (do not try to get somewhere) Imagine that each step you make is making you more and more peaceful.

Chapter Six: Your Meditation Practice

Step 7: Feel the ground, be fully aware of where and how you are stepping. Step fully (from heel to toe).

Your Sacral Chakra

Your Sacral Chakra is called Swaadhisthhaan. It is located in the area of the spine that is aligned with your ovaries or testes. This Chakra is associated with sex, creation and the water element. So creativity, joy and enjoyment of your five senses are associated with this Chakra. Being able to "go with the flow" of life will increase when your sacral Chakra is balanced.

Once you are feeling secure in this world (your root Chakra is balanced) you need to master your emotions and ability to enjoy life. If you are stressed, you do not take the time to find joy and pleasure in your life. Any kind of change leaves you reeling and you feel like life is a "daily grind".

How to balance your Sacral Chakra

I will make a few suggestions to open and balance your sacral Chakra. Again, these are just guidelines; if you have other rituals to connect you with your senses and sensual self, go for it. The intention of these exercises is to increase your capacity for joy and enjoyment.

- Belly dancing
- Surround yourself with things that you find joyful, fun and beautiful (flowers, art, sculpture)

Your Peace Diet

- Spending time near a body of water (a rain puddle does not count!)

- Engaging in your five senses what is your favorite Smell? Taste? Sound? Texture?

- Do something fun and spontaneous

- Again you may use affirmations such as "I nourish my spirit", "Pleasure is a divine part of my life" and "I am creative"

Flower Gazing

It is said that one of Mahatma Buddha's sermons was to hold a flower up to the audience in silence. He had a twinkle in his eye as he twirled it.

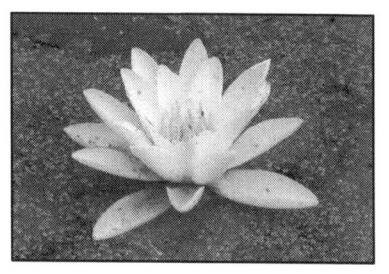

This sermon enlightened Mahakashyapa, the founder of Zen.

Let us also see if we can find joy and insight by recreating that sermon.

- Sit crossed-legged or comfortably in a chair.

- Take any flower that attracts you and hold it in your hand.

Chapter Six: Your Meditation Practice

- Notice the fragile petals, the beautiful color and fragrance.

- Reflect on its beauty and that its value is all about the beauty it gives to the world.

- Contemplate that enjoying the physical world and the pleasures it gives does not make you a hedonist as long as you are living in balance.

Remember, your Chakras are just indications of the energy that you are putting out into the world. Make sure that you are fulfilling all of your needs in this world including time for pleasure, relaxation and relationships.

Are you having trouble with being joyful? Is being worried or anxious still overriding your ability to seek pleasure? The next chapter explores your emotions and what you can do to master them.

CHAPTER SEVEN: THE EMOTIONAL PLANE – BATTLING YOUR FEELINGS

Despite trying to repress them, suppress them and deny them, emotions are a vital part of who we are and why we do the things we do.

There is a negative connotation to being called "emotional". It is almost the same as being called insane. Yet everyone has emotions.

Marketing 101 claims that most people buy with their emotions and then use their logic to explain why the purchase was a good one. This shows that emotion still plays a large part in our lives.

So what do we do about our emotions? In this section we look at how your emotions are related to your stress levels, what Eastern philosophies say about the cause of unhappiness and how to cultivate emotions that help you with your peace diet.

Chapter Seven: The Emotional Plane – Battling with your feelings

Emotions and Stress

There are two things that we need to work on to remove the stress and anxiety build up that happens. One is that because our society looks at emotions negatively and that we bottle it up inside, we stop recognizing emotions. Your body then starts displaying physical symptoms. Such as

- Pains and Headaches
- Fatigue
- Stomach trouble
- Muscle and joint stiffness.

The second thing that most stress and anxiety comes from is a place of fear. Fear, not sadness is the killer of our happiness. Most of our fears come from

- Fear of losing our jobs/money
- Fear for our safety
- Fear of losing love
- Fear of losing respect
- Fear of you or your loved ones dying

You need to recognize first what is going on inside your body, learn about the emotions and thoughts that are there. It won't be pleasant at first, you will be surprised at the amount of negative things you tell yourself and the things that you don't want to have happen because you are afraid, but having the courage (yes, you are being brave because most people do not want to look inside themselves) to do this will help you enormously.

Apathy or the inability to feel

Most of us in the Western world are suffering with this disease. We have no idea how we are feeling and most of us are neither interested nor excited about life and living. Most of us go about our lives like we are robots. We have our routines that we stick to, the expectations and roles that we need to fulfill and the occasional splurge on something that fits into one or more of the above expectations. This is why so many of us have affairs, or mid-life crises. Those things allow us to shake off the apathy for a while. I am not in any way condoning these practices but if we learned to accept our emotions and if we didn't look at emotions as being so horrible, we might avoid these behaviors altogether. So step one on this journey? Let's find out what emotions are locked inside you right now.

Witnessing your emotions

You must first learn to recognize and then witness your emotional state. The only way to do that is to do a session of Zen meditation. Zen comes from the Chinese word Chan, which comes from the word Dhyaana or contemplation.

Chapter Seven: The Emotional Plane – Battling with your feelings

Dhyaana is one of the eight limbs of Patanjali, who organized yoga into what it is today.

Here is my suggestion for witnessing your emotions:

Emotion Watching Meditation (10-15 mins)

Sit in a comfortable position, either on the floor or a straight back chair. If you are in a chair put both feet on the ground and put your hands on your lap.

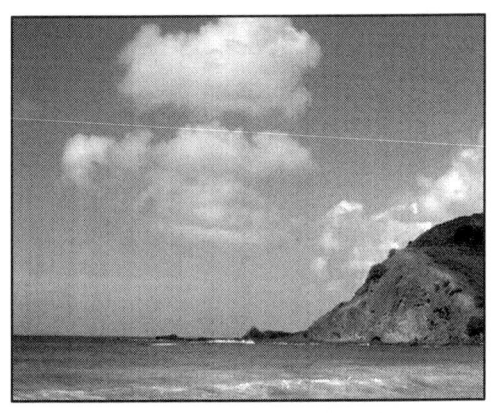

You are going to imagine that you are looking up into a blue sky. It is a beautiful color with white, fluffy clouds.

Soon, a thought is going to come into your head. Think of it floating away into the blue sky the way a balloon would.

After you have sent a few balloons away (quite a few in my case) something else begins to arrive. It does not seem to come as a thought, but as a sensation in your body.

Tune into that sensation. Where in your body is it?

See if you can identify the emotion. Do you feel sad, happy, angry, afraid? Something more complex?

Your Peace Diet

Stay with this sensation in your body. Now see if you can see it. What color is it? Does it move? Put some space between you and the sensation. Look at that sensation the way you would look at something in a glass box.

Now imagine sending love to that sensation and let it out of the box. Allow it to pass through your body and out through the ground.

Do this as many times as you must until you feel empty and light.

Don't be surprised if nothing shows up the first time you do this. Keep on trying, because knowing what emotions you have inside you is half the battle.

The Battle with Fear

Most of our stress and anxiety is linked in some way to a fear that we have. Another way to say this is that we are always worried (another form of fear) about a problem that we have. We think: I would be happy if only (insert problem here) was solved.

So how do we fight off fear? How do we stop worrying about our problems? Remember, if you stop worrying you will be removing a deep-seated root of your stress and anxiety. Imagine what your life would be like if you worried less. No, no, don't go into "I would be happy if only I worried less...." Worrying is a bit self-perpetuating isn't it?

Chapter Seven: The Emotional Plane – Battling with your feelings

Well lucky for you I have two emotions that you can use like a bullet proof vest against worry shooting at you constantly. Here they are:

Gratitude

Ah yes, there have been books about it. Self-help gurus have raved about it and if you are religious, sermons have spoken about the virtues of this emotion. Tell me something I don't know, you're thinking. Yes, I know you know about gratitude. I just have one question.

Are you grateful every day?

I'm must admit I don't formally practice this every day, but it's when I focus on this emotion that I'm not afraid anymore. I remember how many good things I have in my life and I am filled with happiness. And happiness trumps fear. It is this thought that you must have to block out worry which leads to anxiety which leads to stress and we've talked about how bad stress is for you already.

Appreciation

This is not the same as gratitude. Appreciation is when you actively express your gratitude. You tell people thank you for being there for you, for giving you support, for making you laugh? Expressing gratitude is even more powerful as it allows those good feelings to be shared with others. And boy does that feel even better!

Your Peace Diet

Stop reading now and make a list of ways you can be:

- Grateful everyday

- Thank others for how much they have helped you everyday

Make this a daily part of your peace diet and you'll never have to battle your emotions again. Well maybe not as much.

Desires and the Bhagwad Geeta

Eastern philosophy believes that much of our suffering comes from our desires. It states that if you can have equanimity, you would have achieved true peace of mind and enlightenment. I remember being told that being able to look at gold and a rock as the same, a beautiful woman as your sister or daughter (obviously this saying was for men!) and to smile when others insult you was to be a true sage or Rishi.

Now, as my husband pointed out, there seems to be a few flaws in this thinking. Desire is the motivation to do anything in life and if you do not desire anything then staying home in bed all day would make you enlightened.

This is where I remember the words of the *Bhagwad Geeta* or the "Song Divine". A little background first. The Geeta (or Gita) is a part of a larger historical epic called the Mahabharata. The Mahabharata is not considered a religious text, but a historical account.

Chapter Seven: The Emotional Plane – Battling with your feelings

The *Geeta* begins near the end of the epic. I'll do a quick recap so you can get your bearings. Once upon a time there were two bands of brothers. These bands were cousins. One band was called the Kauravas and the other was the Pandavas. They were fighting over a large kingdom their fathers had left them.

When the *Geeta* begins, the Kauravas have usurped the kingdom through deceit and stealth. After much political negotiation, the Kauravas still declare war. All of Bhagavan Krishna's (an incarnation of Vishnu) efforts for peace have been refused. Krishna refuses to take arms, but agrees to act as a charioteer for the legendary archer Arjun. Arjun's army is relying on his strength to win this battle.

Arjun loses his will to fight when he goes off to the middle of the battlefield and sees all of his relatives on the opposing side of the battle field.

Bhagavan Krishna begins to appease him by reminding him of his duties. In one of the more famous quotes Bhagavan Krishna says:

"You have a right to act but not a right to the fruits of your action. Therefore, do not act in anticipation of the fruit yet do not succumb to inaction."

Many people interpret this quote (remember this already has lost some of its original meaning because it has been translated) to mean that we should not desire anything. You should just go about your life without wanting or needing anything.

I have a slightly different interpretation. I think that you should be motivated, a spark of desire is needed to start a journey or you would not get anywhere. I had the desire to share what I have learned about Yoga with a larger audience, so I am writing this book. If I didn't have that desire, you would not be reading this book now.

And remember not having the "right" just means that you do not have the control. It doesn't mean that if something is successful you cannot enjoy it.

But, you must let go of the attachment to the outcome and get enjoyment from the journey.

Are you enjoying your journey?

CHAPTER EIGHT: THE MENTAL PLANE – YOUR MYTHS AND LEGENDS

We are diving deep into the root causes of your stress and anxiety now. We're heading into your mental plane, the part of you that's in charge of your thoughts. Those initial sparks and chemical reactions create your world.

It sounds really "out there" doesn't it? But think about it. Let's look at this idea on a very simple level. You're brushing your teeth in the morning and you realize you're running out of toothpaste. You think, "I need to get more toothpaste at the grocery" and of course you act on that thought. Sooner or later.

Here's a more complex idea. You are browsing online and you notice a new product. It is has very good reviews, and the appeal of a new iPad. You think wow, I'd love that! But it's too expensive and you go back to your work. A few weeks later you get some mail (virtual or otherwise) saying SALE! Get 30% OFF.... and the product you wanted is staring back at you in

Technicolor. You think, hey maybe I'll just go check it out, and then, before you know it, you're back home, excited as a five year-old with your new toy. Oh and some other things that were on sale that you really needed.

Your thoughts create your world

Can you see now on a very practical level how your thoughts begin to create your world? Can you think about how this works with friendships? Relationships? Your job or career? A thought led you to deciding to buy and read this book, right? So let's look break this down a little more.

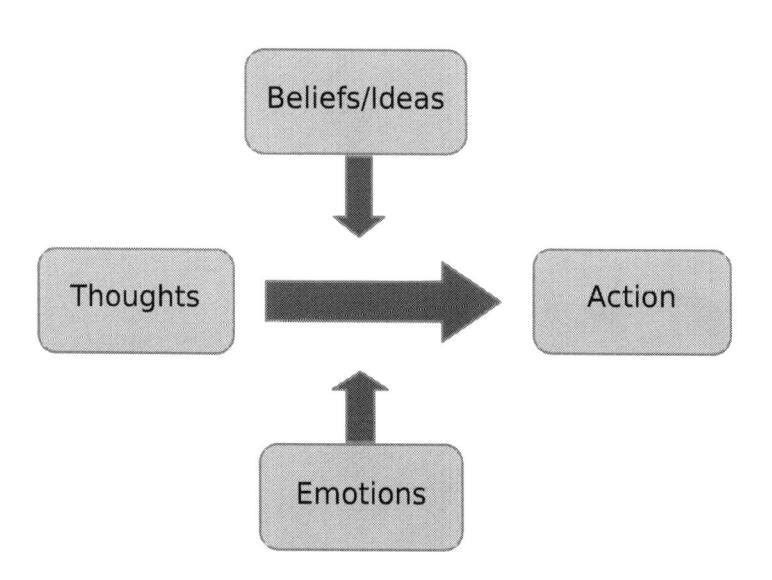

```
        Beliefs/Ideas
              |
              v
Thoughts  ========>  Action
              ^
              |
          Emotions
```

Chapter Eight: The Mental Plane – Your Myths and Legends

Step 1: You have a thought. Now this can be caused by seeing something, a conversation or some external or internal stimuli.

Step 2: This thought is mixed with how you feel about your thought as well as your previous ideas or beliefs.

Step 3: The thought mixed with your emotions, beliefs and ideas cause you to act. I count inaction as a form of "action" so not doing something shapes your world as much as doing something.

For example, you own a small business and you've been invited to a network meeting. Now, not going will have as much of an impact on your business as going.

Your Problems

So what is a problem anyway? Let's think about problems in general. They fall into one of two categories.

Things that you wish would happen and **Things you wish weren't happening or will not happen.**

That's it!

So it's either a desire that hasn't been fulfilled or a fear of something that either is happening or may happen in the future.

Your Peace Diet

This is why so many Eastern philosophies say that desires cause suffering. If you did not have the desire for something, you would not be suffering.

I know all about this problem. I've battled with it myself on many occasions. Let's take for example a woman who can't have children.

Many women are facing trouble with fertility and if you're one of them, this world can be a difficult place to live in. Some women who are having trouble conceiving can't even look at children.

Even though I understand, I feel that these women are being unfair to themselves. By making your desire overwhelm your life you are caging yourself. Your desire will indirectly dictate things like places you can and can't go, friendships you can make or have to break because of children and events that may have children.

You turn from a functioning human being into a victim.

Wishing something wasn't true is an even more direct route to victimhood. How many times have you told yourself "I don't have money, a partner, a better job"? Remember everyone has been subject to hurtful behavior, legal or financial issues, or health-related problems.

There is a difference between going through a difficult time and acting like a victim of life.

Chapter Eight: The Mental Plane – Your Myths and Legends

Now, before we go on to discuss victimhood, I would like to say two things.

First I am not dictating these solutions to you from on high, having overcome all of these issues.

These ideals are more like climbing up a sand dune. Each step is slippery and you can easily slide or even have a huge fall and have to begin the climb again. I have fallen many times and I am still learning how to stop acting and feeling like a victim.

That being said, understanding these principles are easy, having the courage to act on them over and over again is hard. If you continue to climb, things will get clearer. I'm just holding out my hand to you for you to get your footing.

Victimhood

Everyone faces times where they are wronged or facing a challenge. How we perceive ourselves during these times though will lead us out into a completely different future.

A victim mindset leads to:

- inaction
- fear
- anger
- negative habits

For example, when June was little, her mother and father used to fight constantly. Her parents divorced. They did not get along even after the divorce and the joint custody. June could look at herself as a product of divorce. She feels that there is "something wrong with her" and that plays out in her relationships with men. She can never seem to stay in a relationship for long.

A positive mindset leads to:

- action
- gratitude
- getting help

June could also look at the divorce as positive. Her parents decided that being in an unhappy and unsatisfying relationship was a bad example for her. She could then ask them about what happened, continue to be close and understanding to both people and even use those lessons to avoid getting into difficult relationships.

The same event looks different from different mindsets and has very different outcomes. Even in the most difficult circumstances, a positive mindset is a better road to follow.

Chapter Eight: The Mental Plane – Your Myths and Legends

The Pollyana Syndrome

Of course, backlash to positive thinking says that positive thinkers live in a fantasy world and they are unaware of reality (this would be something my sister would say to me often). They call it the Pollyana Syndrome based on novel and movie *Pollyana*. Realists believe that realism is the only way to truly view the world as it is. I am not going to argue with this. All I am going to ask is, are you interested in being right or getting results? I am not asking you to "make believe" anything with positive thinking but you can tell a story two ways.

Your life, who you are and what has happened is a story that you tell over and over in your head. This dictates what you do, what you believe and how you act. I would like you to take some time and write your life story. Focus on the problems you had, bad situations you found yourself in, the things that you wish you did but didn't.

Finished?

Look at the story as if you were a complete stranger and ask yourself these questions. Be brutally honest.

- Would you like to meet this person?

- Would you feel this person brings value to the world?

Now, rewrite your story. Focus on the problems that you solved or difficult circumstances you overcame. Maybe a dream you fulfilled.

Ask the same questions again. I'm sure the answers are quite different. One last question: did you lie about yourself in either story?

New myths and legends

Our life stories that we carry around in our heads are our myths and legends. We carry around myths and legends that are larger than life, tragedies or happy endings.

Think about your positive myths and legends. Maybe it is a story about your family. During family gatherings it usually starts off with "Remember the time…?" Do those stories empower you or embarrass you? Can you think about ways to emphasize the positive myths and legends?

What about your personal myth, the story that you tell yourself? I've already had you write your positive personal myth. Now I would like you to add your personal fairy tale ending. What would your best outcome be?

Visualization

The next thing on the mental plane that can aggravate stress and anxiety or soothe it is your vision for the future. So many self-help books tell you that you need "positive visualization"

Chapter Eight: The Mental Plane – Your Myths and Legends

tools to make you rich or help you lose weight or to fix the problem that you are having. So many people complain that they "can't visualize" and it is too hard.

What they fail to realize is that they already visualizing. They are very good at it and do it easily, but they do it in the form of worry, anxiety and fear.

The complaint really is, "I can only visualize negative things, and how do I change that?" Again, this seems to be our set point. We all automatically tune in to the negative and we have to work on visualizing the positive. This was good when we were hunters and gatherers because it helped us to survive, but now it just holds us back. So what to do?

Well, instead of trying to visualize you need to focus on your **Feelings First.**

Continue to use tools to make you aware of how you feel (see chapter 7 for the *Witnessing Emotions Meditation*). When you can tune into positive emotions more than negative ones, then you are ready to start visualizing positive outcomes in your life.

Also do something real. Schedule that meeting, go to that party. Positive planning increases your chances for positive visualizations.

Here's an example. Let's say you're worried about money, you just don't seem to have enough. Witness your emotions surrounding money and when you can start to feel positive about money, start to track down to the penny all of the money flowing **into** your life.

If you are feeling even more positive you can even plan a budget, but don't try it when you are worried. Remember positive feelings first!

Responsibility vs. Fate: The Bhagvad Geeta revisited

Even though I have written a lot on taking responsibility for your thoughts, feelings and actions, when it comes to stress and anxiety, I feel that in some cases, stress and anxiety are caused by trying to control things which we have no control over. And we mistake control for responsibility.

We worry about natural disasters, about the weather about the safety of grown children. We worry about how people will react or treat us; we worry about getting ill and dying.

Part of the *Serenity Prayer* by Reinhold Niebuhr states...

... grant me the serenity
to accept the things I cannot change;
courage to change the things I can;
and wisdom to know the difference.

Living one day at a time;
Enjoying one moment at a time;
Accepting hardships as the pathway to peace.

Chapter Eight: The Mental Plane – Your Myths and Legends

I believe that part of the reason that stress is so prevalent in our modern world is because we feel that we can control everything in our lives. Our ancestors did not feel they were in control of everything. If something happened to them, it was "fate". Rubs you the wrong way doesn't it. But we've gone completely the other way. Take Karma for instance.

A side effect of believing in karma is that revenge doesn't happen as often. Many people, after they are hurt by someone, don't feel it's important to exact revenge. "They will get what is coming to them," these people say when they've been hurt. This allows you to forgive, forget and move on more easily than if you believe that the person needs to feel pain and you must be the person to deliver that pain.

So even if the Law of Karma is not true, just like positive thinking, which one looks like the healthier option?

With this new piece of information, the verse in the Bhagwad Geeta takes on new meaning:

"You have a right to act but not a right to the fruits of your action. Therefore, do not act in anticipation of the fruit yet do not succumb to inaction."

If you act and enjoy your actions, without even thinking about the outcome, then will your worry and stress be higher or lower? Will you feel the need to control things? Remember to enjoy your life, the process and the journey. Remember to feel both the good and the bad. Don't get so focused on the destination that you forget to look out the window and see what you're passing by.

You're nearing the end of your yoga journey. You have peeled of layer after layer and come to the center of yourself. Your consciousness, life spark or soul. In the final chapter, we will talk about what you can do to ensure that your soul is fed and how your soul manifests in the physical world.

CHAPTER NINE: THE SPIRITUAL PLANE – YOUR CONSCIOUSNESS AND HOW YOU VIEW THE WORLD

We've come from the physical world, a world of senses, to the world of being. Let's start off with a story, shall we?

There is a very strange tale from the Upanishads that I was told as a young girl. Here it is and my interpretation of it. Yours may be different.

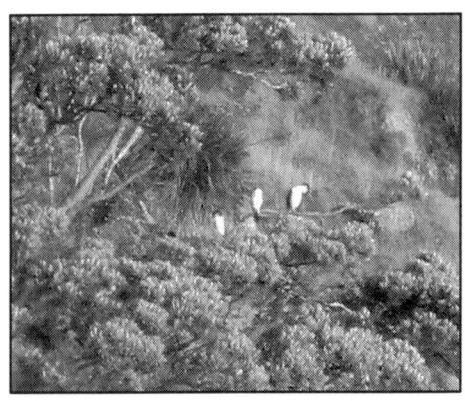

Once there were two birds sitting on a tree. They were inseparable friends. One bird would wander around the tree restlessly and finally finding a berry it would eat the berry. The second bird would just watch. When it is finished the first bird would go off to find another berry. The second bird would look on at the first bird. Doing nothing but witnessing its actions.

Now as a girl I thought it was strange. Why didn't the first bird give the second bird a berry? Didn't the second bird get hungry? Obviously I didn't understand the idea of symbolism.

The first bird is your mind. Always active, restless, always searching for pleasure in one place or another. The second bird is your consciousness or your being. It sits and observes, being a witness to life. It is always constant and true.

Many times this story is also told to describe the difference between the Atman or human soul and the Paramatman or supreme soul. The Paramatman is the divinity within each person according to one philosophy or God according to another.

If you think about it, you can recall a time where you feel that you are not "feeling" things, you are just observing things. The positive side of this is what artists and athletes call being "in the flow".

The negative side is when a person experiences terrible trauma like a crash or a near death experience.

Eckhart Tolle gives yet another example when he reflects on his despair and suicidal thoughts in, *The Power of Now*. He asks

Chapter Nine: The Spiritual Plane – Your Consciousness

"am I one or two? If I cannot live with myself, there must be two of me: the 'I' and the 'self' that 'I' cannot live with."

Even if you don't believe you have a soul, you can understand that there seems to be duality in our minds and consciousness. It is this part of you that usually concerns you the least. After all, it's always there. But this is also the part of you that you need to care for the most because if you nurture it will determine the fitness of your physical, mental and emotional makeup.

So how do we go about feeding our souls, the very essence of our being?

Experiencing the sacred in daily life

My husband enjoys washing dishes. At first, I just couldn't understand. How could he be so enthusiastic about dishes? I dislike doing them with a passion. Well, one day he told me his secret. He said if you learned to find joy in doing what most of us consider "work" you will find much more joy in your life. Pretty philosophical for a computer guy, mathematician and engineer.

I am not going to ask you to try to do that. I think we'll save that for an advanced session on the art of living. What I will ask you to take a look at is how much time do you devote to doing something that does not have a goal?

Your Peace Diet

This goes beyond disconnecting. For many of you, switching off your phone, computer, radio and television seems distressing but I'm going to go even further and suggest that what you decide to do must accomplish nothing, get you nowhere and cause absolutely no effort in you at all.

You see, I can give you a list of things for you to choose to nurture your spirit, but you can create goals for things like meditating, yoga, reading and watching television if you're not careful. Even going for a walk can have a goal. So let's focus on this instead: What can you do that is extremely pleasurable and that has no goal?

There are two main ways that you can tell whether what you are doing is goal free:

Connectedness: You feel connected, whether it is to a person or people, or to something more abstract like nature or the universe (when have you looked up at the stars or the moon lately?)

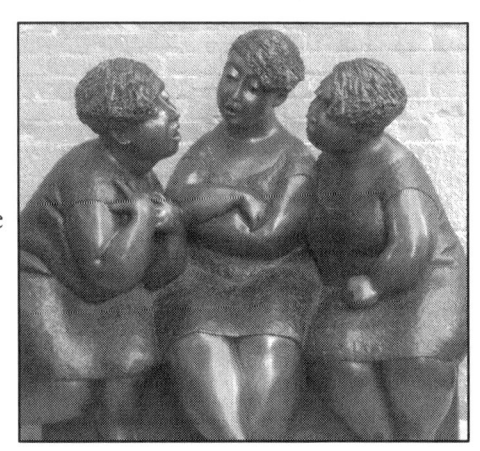

Presence: You feel completely in the present moment. You've forgotten about the pressing meeting that's making you nervous

Chapter Nine: The Spiritual Plane – Your Consciousness

or the never ending list of things that you have to do. All you were thinking of was being right in that moment.

Keeping these two things in mind I am going to ask you to find a way to be in that state for at least 10 minutes each day. This is an absolute "must". Here are "ideas" for you:

- sit in a garden
- go star gazing or cloud gazing
- sing out loud to your favorite song (it doesn't matter that you're tone deaf!)
- stare into space
- if you have pets, pet them; if you don't have pets borrow someone else's
- listen to music
- go out with a friend for a chat
- pray or meditate
- spend time in nature (it's scientific name: Attention Restoration Theory)

As Above, So below

Paulo Coelho refers to this phrase in his book *The Alchemist*. The Law of Attraction craze is based on this. But what does it mean? Let me tell you another story that was told to me often as a girl.

Once there was an old innkeeper whose inn was located between two major cities. One traveler asked "I'm on my way to the other city, can you tell me what it's like there?"

The innkeeper replies, "Tell me what it was like in the previous city."

"I enjoyed my stay very much. The people were generous and friendly. It was clean and bright and the food that was served was delicious."

"The other city is like that also," said the innkeeper.

After a while another traveler came to stay at the inn. He also was going the same way and asked about the next city.

The innkeeper asked him the same question.

"Oh it was terrible," replied the man, "the people were mean and unfriendly. The city was cold, and the meals were disgusting."

"The other city is like that also," said the innkeeper.

Chapter Nine: The Spiritual Plane – Your Consciousness

Two people were in the same city at the same time and had vastly different experiences. How is that even possible?

Well I had this happen to me firsthand. I was on a tour of Europe and we had stopped for a day in Paris. I had a wonderful time. I thought that most of the people were friendly and kind; the city was warm and beautiful and full of culture. Of course I tried to communicate the best that I could in French.

That evening a few of my fellow tourists were discussing Paris and to my shock they had an awful day! They were treated badly, they thought the city was dangerous with the traffic and crowds and they just wanted to go home.

How could such a thing happen?

Both stories illustrate that you create your own experiences, by how you see the world. (Trying to speak French also helped in my case).

Your very being crafts how you perceive the world and therefore what happens in it. This is not a perfect outcome and again sounds like a bunch of New Age mumbo jumbo, but you have had this happen to you too. Here's an example:

You've just bought a new car (or shirt or iPad), and suddenly it seem to be popping up everywhere. Did everyone buy a car like yours all of a sudden? Probably not, but it has now become a focus for your attention.

Your Peace Diet

The same thing happens with your life outlook. If you are consistently grumpy and complaining, you'll find more things to be grumpy and complain about. If you are happy, you'll find more things to be happy about.

Changing who you are is not easy. It is possible, but not easy. So many ideas like the Law of Attraction book *The Secret* makes it sound so simple. Change your thinking and you'll get rich, have great relationships and have a great life. All you need to do is read the book and watch the movie.

Changing your thoughts means changing your being and that takes a lot of work.

Gosh that sounds just like doom and gloom doesn't it? The main thing that I'm trying to tell you is that you shouldn't be so hard on yourself.

No program, book or movie will be able to make a lasting change. Not unless you've put in a lot of work. So don't feel like a failure if you have been thinking "I'm a millionaire" and nothing has happened. It takes more than that to become a millionaire. It takes learning the skills you need to become a millionaire. It takes looking every day at the things that you are doing to bring you closer to that goal. It takes you showing up day after day with the same enthusiasm that you started with at Day 1.

Chapter Nine: The Spiritual Plane – Your Consciousness

Sound too hard? What if I told you that you've done this already? More than once in your life? I could guarantee that at least 95% of you reading this book have pursued a goal with as much passion despite all the odds.

What was it that you showed up enthusiastically day after day until you mastered it?

Walking and talking. This was a near impossible goal as a baby. It took tireless effort, day after day, but you did it. Remember that when you feel that changing your reality isn't going as well as you'd want it.

Change is hard, but have the courage to try.

Living with Integrity

This is so important that I've saved it for last. You are a unique fingerprint in the world. So many people try to fit themselves into a physical, mental and spiritual mold.

Part of the reason so many people feel that their lives need fixing are because they don't appreciate themselves – the unique beings that they are.

Do you really need to change who you are to get that new job, new boyfriend, new house or to influence how others think of you?

Your Peace Diet

Living with Integrity simply means that deciding who you are is amazing. This doesn't mean that you cannot set goals and do things, but it means that these goals come from deep within you. It is there to please only you, not anyone else.

Does it sound like you're being selfish? You're not. Connecting with people and helping others is something that gives me deep pleasure. Those who I've helped know that I didn't do it out of obligation, or to look good, they know I helped because I wanted to and they're probably grateful for that.

It also brings me deep joy if I can find circumstances that will bring what's called a win-win situation. I believe that there are ways to conduct business, work and relationships that gives value to everyone concerned.

When you decide to do things that align with your unique self and step into that then things become easier. The roads "rise up to meet you".

Living with integrity makes the very things we talked about at the beginning of the book, your body, your environment, your thoughts, habits and emotions easier to manage.

Live with the ability to be authentic and do what you say you will do. Be who you say you will be. After all, that's why you are here. You are a unique tree with your roots interconnecting with the forest. You are a wave in the ocean. Unique yet joined deeply to the vastness of the sea and the world.

Chapter Nine: The Spiritual Plane – Your Consciousness

You were born to be who you are. Make all of your choices with that in mind. Do what you are and you will begin to realize that this will help you to achieve your goals with ease, without stress, anxiety and with much peace.

I am pleased to have walked a short way with you on your journey through life. There is an Indian saying that "if you walk seven steps together with a stranger, you become friends".

Namaste my friend,

Lakshmi Gosyne

For more information or help with *Your Peace Diet* please visit www.newbieyoga.com, or contact me at newbieyogateam@newbieyoga.com. If you would like support with making the changes outlined in the book, we can help you at www.newbieyoga.com/our-services

ABOUT THE AUTHOR

Yoga and meditation have been a part of my life since I was a little girl. I learned poses off and on for many years, but focused more on martial arts instead.

Then, a crazy thing happened to me. I fell in love and moved to New Zealand. Within a year I was halfway around the world. Moving countries is exciting but can take a toll on you.

I started meditating because I felt very lost. I took the ten-day Vipassana Course in Kaukapakapa to get some perspective on my life. I learned a lot about meditation, but I found it difficult to practice the proper Vipassana meditation for two hours every day. I now meditate by listening to some meditation music to get me to relax and then silent meditation.

I started my daily yoga practice because I was diagnosed with unexplained infertility. At first I started Iyengar classes, and it was very informative, but I'm a bit of an introvert so I currently practice at home.

Qualifications:

Bachelor's Degree in Psychology

Bachelor's Degree in Classical Indian Music (from BVS)

Master's Degree in Education

Second Degree Black Belt in Taekwondo

Green Belt in Kiaido Ryu

Meditation Teacher Certification.

Made in the USA
Charleston, SC
09 August 2011